York
Abdominal
Course

Bob Hoffman

ISBN: 149616993X
ISBN-13: 978-1496169938

CONTENTS

1   Culture of the Abdomen

2   Abdominal Culture

3   24 Splendid Exercises

4   12 Exercises with Weights

5   Better Health Through Overcoming Obesity

6   Abdominal Course Exercise Chart

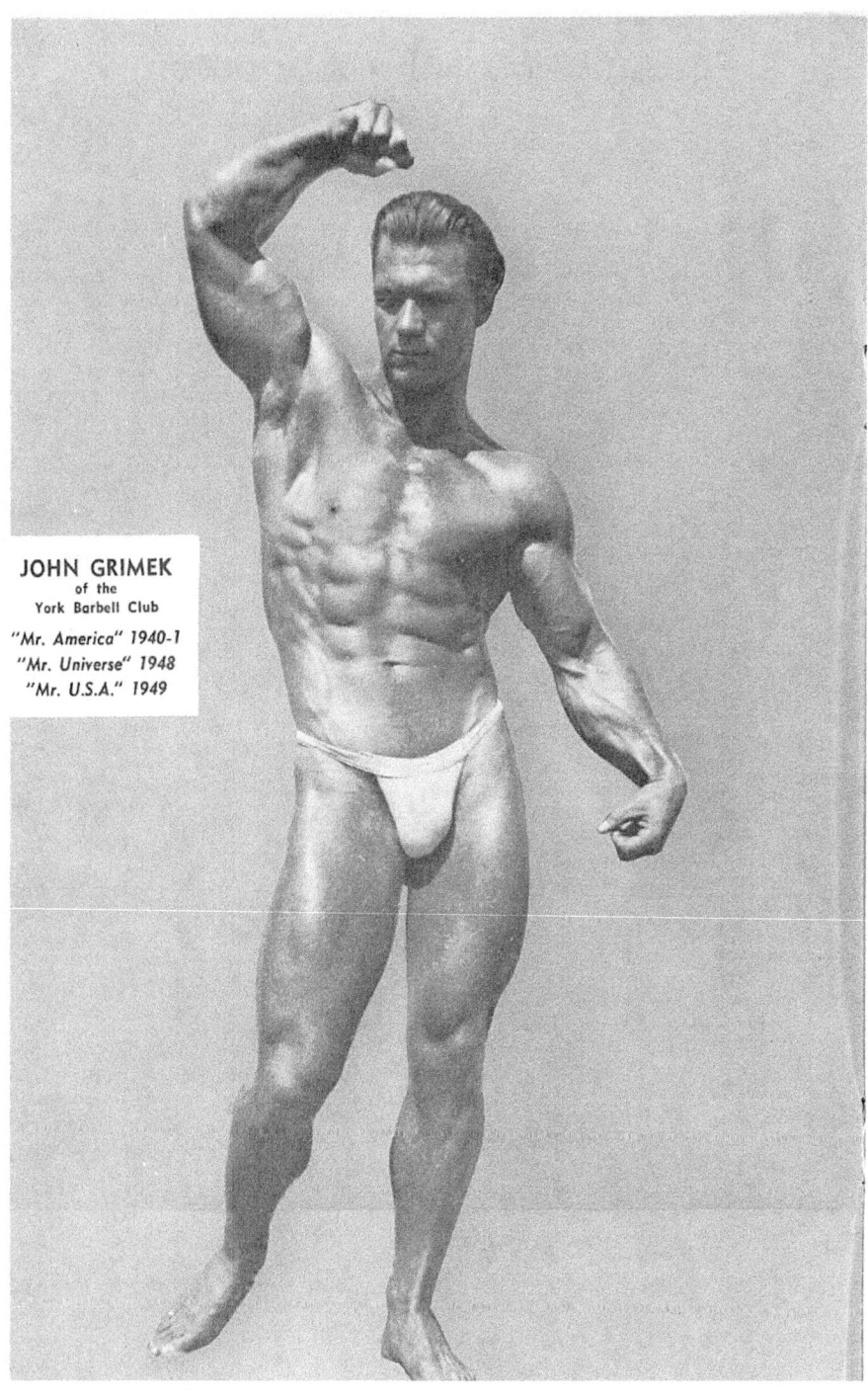

JOHN GRIMEK
of the
York Barbell Club

"Mr. America" 1940-1
"Mr. Universe" 1948
"Mr. U.S.A." 1949

Culture of the Abdomen

By BOB HOFFMAN

U. S. Olympic Coach

THE most important muscles of the body and also the most neglected are the muscles of the mid section. These include the abdominal muscles and the muscles of the lower back and sides. The vast majority of civilized people do not exercise the muscles of the mid section at all and even those who follow exercise programs of various sorts, rarely, if at all, perform special exercises for the mid section. The muscles of the limbs, particularly the arms, receive the Lion's share of attention in the majority of exercise programs. Light exercise systems invariably include innumerable arm and shoulder exercises. Too often more advanced methods of training with elastic exercisers of all sorts, dumbell training with flat or inclined bench and pulley exercisers do not include a single side or abdominal developing exercise. The courses most body builders follow are usually designed only to build the muscles of the extremities, with little thought given to building internal or organic strength with the super health which is sure to accompany it.

We have always believed in the axiom that any exercise is better than no exercise but to obtain the most from your physical training you should follow a good all around program designed to develop all the important muscles of the body, particularly the mid section. Too many body builders are interested only in developing muscles which look good, which attract favorable attention with little thought to the practical use of these super developed muscles or of the building of vital power. We spend our lives here at York urging people to make progressive training with graded resistance, barbells, dumbells, swingbells, elastic exercisers, a part of their lives. We constantly urge all ambitious body builders to do what you should first and then go on to do what one wants to do. And what one should do, regardless of one's ambition, is to practice a good all-

around training program before specializing in developing the arms, chest, shoulders, upper back, latissimus etc. Every York course, the various dumbell, swingbell, and barbell courses, includes some exercises for the midsection. These exercises should never be neglected. For exercises which involve the midsection not only strengthen the muscles which keep your body erect, make you a man instead of a beast, the muscles which hold in place and protect the important organs, glands and processes, the engines of the body, but they stimulate and improve every internal process. And regardless of why you exercise or how you exercise, what you seek to accomplish through exercise, whether your desire is to keep fit in the easiest and quickest possible way, whether you desire the limit in strength and development, whether you want to be a champion weight lifter or a physique contest winner, abdominal exercises should be a part of your training program.

The competitive weight lifter needs abdominal work less than any other. For in lifting very heavy weights overhead the muscles of the mid section are placed in vigorous action as they work with the muscles more directly involved in lifting the weights, serve as balancers or stabilizers in keeping the body erect with heavy weights overhead. All weight lifters have powerful, well muscled mid sections. The muscles are there, but I desire all the lifters in my charge to practice some abdominal movements which bend, twist, massage and activate the abdominal section. For this type of exercise improving every internal process, the digestion, assimilation, elimination, glandular action, build super health and more strength, more lifting power.

There is not a class of humans who do not need plenty of abdominal exercise and those who do not practice regular exercise need it most of all. Since the beginning of written history, including the record of painting and sculpturing, a well muscled mid section has always been admired. Through most of the ages, except for short periods when the Falstaff type was considered a sign of health and prosperity, the world has always admired the comparatively slender, well muscled mid section. Examine any of the masterpieces of the sculptors of long ago and you will see unexcelled muscular development of the mid section. Little effort is required to convince you that you will look better if you trim and develop your abdominal region. You are sure to be the butt of many jokes if you have a generous middle, to phrase it very mildly. You will lose much of the pleasures and satisfactions of life if you waddle along, duck-like, with a heavy load, actually a garbage can, in your abdominal region.

Appearance is important. Men and women who have attractive bodies have the most fun from life, they get the invitations to parties, the best jobs, the best life partners. If you have a trim and muscular mid section you look younger, you are alive, wider awake, have more health, more pep, energy and endurance. The load is light, you have more muscles to carry you around, less to carry, for you are not burdened with ugly, useless, unhealthy fat.

Appearance is important, but most important of all, for your health's sake you need plenty of abdominal exercise. If you have been living a comfortable, sedentary life you need abdominal exercise most of all. The action of all the organs, glands and processes of the body are muscular. These organs, glands and processes depend upon you. They can not exercise themselves. They can not use barbells, swingbells, dumbells, and elastic exercisers. And you, your future and your very life depend upon your organs and internal processes. Your future well being depends upon your stomach and allied organs of the digestive tract. To build strength and muscle you are dependent upon the organs of digestion, assimilation, and to keep well, dependent upon the organs of elimination.

It is your problem to keep your internal organs strong and well, ready and able to do their work well. You are their doctor. They can not come to you and tell you of their aches, pains, troubles and indispositions, when they are not well and happy they have ways of letting you know about it. And most of these ways are not pleasant, and when they complain, you have to subscribe for them. You must take care of them as if they were your children. Their life and their success depend upon you and your success in life, in body building, depends on how they perform for you.

You can't see what is going on within your mid section, but it is constantly taking place just the same. A myriad of muscles are keeping house for you, and you must help them keep things in order. The organs feed, provide fuel, and drive the muscles. And through exercise you improve the functions of these organs. Abdominal exercise not only strengthens the muscles which support the all important organs, but the action engendered by exercise, the rubbing, massaging, squeezing, the internal exercise, improves assimilation, betters metabolism, hastens digestion, causes elimination to be more thorough.

To develop strength and muscle to a high degree it is necessary to develop the organs to a high degree too. Through abdominal exercise one builds a good digestive system which in turn builds big muscles, builds a good Nervous System so it is easier to maintain a tranquil mind, builds a strong, perfectly operating heart and lungs, and below the diaphragm, the huge muscular plate which separates the heart and lungs from the abdominal region, it develops maximum strength and efficiency in all the organs and processes.

It will pay you well to spend some time cultivating your abdomen, for this means cultivating YOU. If you consider just how you are put together you will better see the need for abdominal exercise. In a four legged animal you can visualize the organs like clothes on a line hanging from the back bone. When that animal stood on end and became man, you can picture all of the organs like clothes on a line hanging down to the floor or ground. This would occur were it not for the fact that there is a place for every organ and they are held in that place, normally, by the muscles. But when these muscles soften, weaken, lose their strength and elasticity the organs sag, the stomach and sides bulge, internal fat forms, organic action is greatly hindered and you do not receive the maximum benefit from your organs, for the fat encased organs and glands can not work properly. A vicious circle is set up. Weak

muscles, more fat, more sluggish action, more clogging, indigestion, constipation, gas and finally aches and pains.

All of these difficulties will disappear when you cultivate or activate your abdomen. Fat likes a nice quiet, inactive place to settle down. It loathes, detests, dislikes, hates and shuns activity. So the best way to eliminate fat inside and out, burdensome, health sapping fat, is to form habits of muscular activity designed to exercise your midsection.

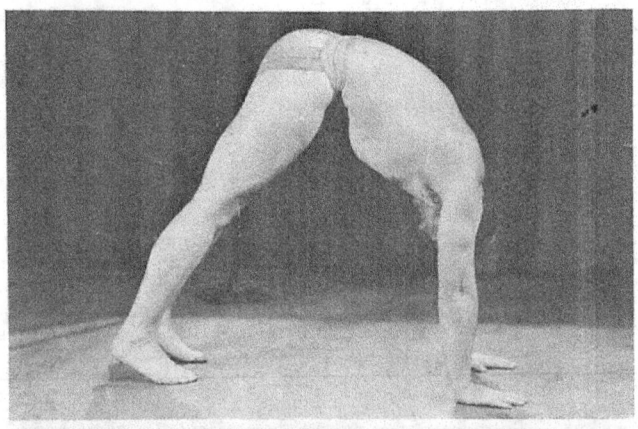

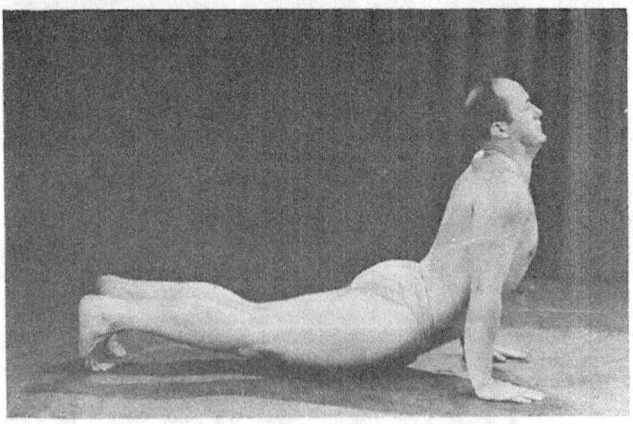

Bob Hoffman, the author, demonstrating exercise No. 5 of the first group in the course. This Hindu exercise is one of the best conditioning movements.

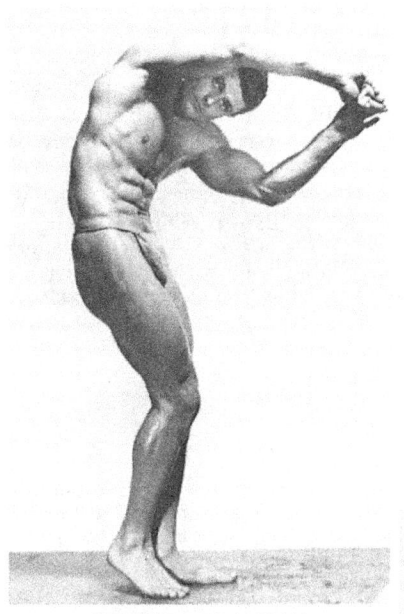

ROBERT DURANTON

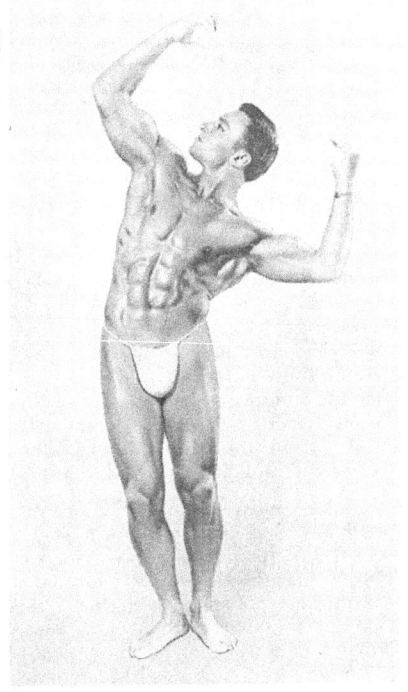

MARVIN URVANT

ABDOMINAL CULTURE

The Abdomen or "mid-section" is the most important part of the body. Here are located many vital organs which control the body's health and well being. The stomach, liver, kidneys, bladder, bowels, intestines, etc., carry on their owner's best interest, in this region.

If you remember something of physiology and anatomy you will know that the muscles hold these organs in place and make it possible for them to perform their functions. I often visualize the organs of four-legged animals as being hung from their backbone like clothes from a line where they have been hung up to dry. The animal finally stood on end and became man. Raise the clothes line on end and the clothes sag into a limp pile. Similarly, man's organs would pile up at the bottom if there were not muscles to hold them in place.

That is why a man who neglects himself physically will finally own a protruding abdomen, a prolapsed stomach, fallen bowels or some other similar condition. It is even worse for a woman as she has more organs.

Fat prefers to form in a nice quiet soft place. A life of ease results in all the organs becoming so coated or surrounded with fat that they perform their vital work sluggishly and with difficulty. Fat does not cling to a strong active muscle. Thus the man who exercises not only has health, but looks and feels youthful regardless of his age.

It has been said that a woman is as old as she looks. A man as old as he feels. This rule works both ways. How you feel and how you look are the two most important things in the world. You can neither look well nor feel well with an out-of shape, bloated, sluggish mid-section. It is not difficult to keep your waist youthful and healthful. Simple rules of exercise. posture and diet will mean a new life for you.

First come simple rules of eating. If your stomach was a powerfully muscled region, strong inside and out, all your bodily processes would work at such high power that you could indulge an appetite like an ostrich or a goat. Strong men can eat or drink vast quantities of most anything without regret. A weak, sick man must watch his food combinations very carefully. Almost count the calories in his food and constantly search for vitamins to be sure that the body receives all the necessary food elements. Various food combinations disagree with some persons. The foods themselves may be quite innocent. But, cotton and glycerine are harmless too. Get them together wih other ingredients and you have "dynamite."

It has been said that "one man's meat is another man's poison." I have always had the most amazing food capacity when I desired to consume a large quantity of foods I liked. During my competitive years when I starred at many forms of athletics my endurance and recuperative powers were considered extraordinary, enough so that I was billed as the "Iron Man" in all athletic competition. I could eat custard pie a la mode with crab cakes, before going to bed and not be disturbed. Many other combinations which were harmful to others were just good food for me. Yet, poached eggs on toast with spinach made me quite ill. They were dynamite to me and disorganized my normally perfect processes, all of which brings out a great truth. "Don't eat things you don't like because you think they are good for you." Eat a wide variety of the foods you like. By this, I do not mean to live on pie, cake, candy and fancy foods, if that is what you like. Try to cultivate the habit of good plain foods; lean meat, preferably beef, mutton, fish or chicken either boiled or roasted than fried. Eat plenty of vegetables. For dessert it is best to eat fresh fruits, preserved fruits, fruit puddings and if you eat pie, make some sort of fruit-pie.

Another most important health rule is to masticate your food thoroughly. Your stomach has no teeth. Strong men eat slowly and deliberately. I don't know whether they are strong men because they eat slowly or whether being strong men they know it is best to eat slowly, but the fact remains, strength and thorough mastication go hand in hand. Chew each bite as long as you can hold it in your mouth. Give it plenty of opportunity to mix with the digestive juices. When drinking liquid, such as milk, sip it. Don't gulp it down. It should be mixed with saliva also.

Eat only at regular mealtimes. This is most important. Cultivate the habit of eating sufficient, to prevent you from becoming too hungry before the next meal. Your stomach is entitled to some rest, too. The digestive process takes from two to six hours, depending on the sort of food eaten and the quantity.
If you eat between meals you spoil your appetite. You have noticed this, haven't you? When the first mouthful of food reaches the stomach, the full load of gastric juices is discharged to start the digestive process. For your stomach does not know whether a full meal is coming or not. And when your regular meal time comes you are not hungry. I know of a young fellow, twelve years old, who had been permitted to nibble at all times, never hungry at meals, so thin his bones almost hurt to touch them. By following these simple rules he gained from 66.5 to 77 pounds in less than four weeks' time. This is a great difference in a small fellow and everyone remarked at how fine he looked these few weeks later.

If you like candy or other sweets eat them immediately after meals only. This is the only time to eat candy or pastries. More complications than you would think arise from always eating. It is a bad habit.
Most persons consume three or four times as much food as they require. If slightly ill or not at all hungry, they "eat to keep their strength up." If you are not hungry, don't eat. If you are really hungry you can easily find out if you are. Think of some plain food and if your mouth waters, you are hungry. Otherwise, it is just a desire for food and you wish to eat because it is twelve or six o'clock.

So many people eat and eat. Get themselves jammed up inside so that the hard-working organs can not clear away the food. Blocked traffic results, just as a heavy snowfall will hold up traffic in a big city until cleared away.
So many people eat only to please their appetite. Highly seasoned, fancy foods, to tempt an appetite that doesn't require food. They should be more concerned about taking good plain foods easily digested and assimilated.

There is a long list of "trash" foods; too long for this short course. Foods that are no more good to the body or no more a source of power than soft mud in the gas tank of your motor. Exercise should not mean constant self-denial. You need not deny yourself everything that you like. But indulge in every-thing with moderation. Any abuse to the body I consider "leaks." Too many "leaks" will sink even a big ship.

Condiments of all sorts—salt, pepper, mustard, catsup, sauces—provide no nourishment for the body. They just tease your appetite. Use them sparingly. Tea and coffee has no food value. White bread, cake, pastries have practically no food value. White sugar has little food value. These and many other foods are just "trash" foods that have to be moved through your system with great effort to your digestive tract. Just as gutters and sewers can be obstructed, your intestines can become clogged. Just as flies collect where there is gar-bage, germs collect when you are overloaded with "trash" foods in your en-tire digestive system. Remove the garbage and the flies disappear. Keep your bowels open and generally clean inside and germs can not collect and you will have finer and greater strength and health.

Constipation comes from wrong foods, upset sluggish organs, wrong eating habits, and lack of exercise. A great many ills come from constipation. Did you ever hear over the radio of the great things that Bug House Water Crystals will do? People have testified that the drinking of this water has cured everything in the line of human ills. It is nothing but salts. It does nothing but partially cleanse your insides. Even finer results would be had by these lazy people if they would eat right and move a little. EXERCISE. They testify to relief from many forms of headaches, bad stomach, bad breath, pimples, boils, lack of energy, gout, and a host of others. All of these could be eliminated just as easily and to a much greater degree—in fact, not experienced at all—with correct eating habits and exercise.

Whether you try to keep fit in two minutes a day by abdominal exercise only or whether you are a seeker of perfect abdominal health and a muscular "wash-board," you will find any and all of the exercises submitted in this course to be most helpful and healthful to you.

A few minutes a day will pay you splendid dividends if spent in abdominal exercise. Cultivate the habit. It will make you rich in health and appearance. This small course contains the 24 best exercises known for the mid-section. They vary from easy, quick, bed-room exercises to heavy work with apparatus, at home or in a gymnasium.

This course has cost you one dollar. One idea you get from it may save you a great many times that amount in the course of your life. In fact it may change the entire course of your life. It is difficult to measure the worth of an idea. It may even mean life to you. Help you build up a fund of health and energy so that you will never experience sickness or pain.

Just one trip to a doctor will cost as much as this course to you. Just a few salts or laxatives will cost you as much. In addition to the information listed here which is the simple and easy way to unusual health and youthful figure, it is your privilege to write to the writer any time, asking for personal advice, instruction or information.

ABDOMINAL CULTURE:

We wish you the best of luck and know you will have it in direct proportion to the effort you put forth and the regularity with which you practice the exercises.

24 SPLENDID EXERCISES

No. 1. I believe this exercise to be the oldest exercise known to man. Certainly it is a good one! You start by standing twenty inches from a wall. Keeping the knees straight and holding the arms overhead, lean back until the arms touch the wall. This stage of the exercise is very good for the small of the back. Leaning back put all the abdominal region into play. Then come forward, touching the floor without bending the knees. Repeat from twelve to twenty-four times.

No. 2. The side-bend is the next exercise. Curl one hand with the palm down over the opposite ear, reaching down as far as you can. At the same time slide the opposite hand as far down the thigh toward or past the knee as you can. Thus you stretch the side muscles to their limit. Leaning first to one side and then the other. Repeating this exercise 12 to 24 times.

No. 3. Lie flat on the floor. Clasp hands back of head. Extend the toes. Keep legs together and hold them straight throughout the exercise. Raise and lower legs steadily and slowly from 12 to 24 times.

No. 4. Stand with the legs 18 inches apart. Hands on hips. While turning as far as you can to the right shoot the arms out horizontally from the side. Then snap back to the center position with hands on hips. Slowly and steadily twist your limit to the opposite side, extending the hands. Snap back to the center, from 12 to 24 times.

No. 5. This exercise is one of the best for the entire mid-section. Place your hands on floor and place your feet as shown in the illustration. You hold the legs quite stiff and arch back as far as possible, pushing with hands and legs. You can see from the illustration of the writer that it is a good exercise. When a 245 pound man can show a waist so slender and a chest so deep it illustrates the worth of this movement. This is one of the Hindu Namaskur exercises which have been practiced since the dawn of history. Originally patterned after the cat tribe's way of keeping fit, they produce marvelous results. Go into the floor-dip position from the starting position. Keeping the legs and hips close to the ground, straighten the arms, bend in the back with considerable force. From this position raise the body into the position shown and described first in this exercise. Repeat this entire sequence of exercises from 12 to 24 times.

No. 6. Stand with the heels together. Raise the arms overhead, turn them so that the fingers lock and are turned palms up. Holding the arms stiff and tight, rotate the body in a circle far to the right, far back, far front. After six entire rotary motions reverse and perform six more the other way, 12 to 24 repetitions for this movement.

No. 7. Lie on your back. Raise the legs to the perpendicular position. Pump them up and down as if you were riding a bicycle. 50 to one hundred movements will not be too many.

ABDOMINAL CULTURE:

No. 8. This exercise is a very simple one. It will serve as a rest between the more strenuous exercises. Simply pull in the stomach as far as you can. Relax and pull it in again, 12 to 24 movements. Get the habit of holding your stomach in, at times while walking, shaving or dressing. You will be pleased with the reduction of your waist line.

No. 9. Sit on bench or box. Place feet under a dresser, weight or strap fastened to floor. Lean back until your extended hands or head touch the floor. Come well forward past the perpendicular position and repeat twelve to twenty-four times.

No. 10. Stand with the feet eighteen inches apart. Reach down and touch the opposite toe with one hand held perpendicularly overhead. Turn your head so that you keep your eyes upon this hand. Come back to the original position, hands on hips. Repeat six to twelve times with each arm, making 12 to 24 times in all.

No. 11. Stand with the feet eighteen inches apart. Permitting the knees to bend slightly with both hands reach far back between legs. Then overhead and back. Do this exercise rapidly 12 to 24 times.

No. 12. Lie on your back. Raise legs, bringing them up and over until they touch the floor back of head. Back to flat position and then repeat to twenty-four times.

12 EXERCISES WITH WEIGHTS: FOR ADVANCED ABDOMINAL CULTURISTS

No. 1. Abdominal raise with bar back of neck. Hold the feet down with weight or strap. Holding bar back of head, keeping legs stiff sit up and go well forward, six to twelve times.

No. 2. Hold fairly heavy dumbell in each hand. Lean slowly as far to the right as possible. Then snap back to center, then lean far to the left. Repeat this exercise 6 to 12 times to each side; 12 to 24 in all.

No. 3. Tie bar bell plates or light dumbells to feet. This to make the exercise progressive so that you can constantly improve the strength and appearance of your abdomen. The York Iron Boots would be suitable for this purpose. Raise and lower the legs, keeping them stiff, keeping the hands under your buttocks to help you maintain the position. Six to twelve times.

No. 4. Take a light dumbell in either hand. Starting with the hands at the side, turn slowly to right, as far as possible, at the same time extend the arms as was done with Exercise No. 4, of the exercises without apparatus. The only difference in this exercise is the fact that more rapid and better results will be had by gradually increasing the weight of the dumbells.

No. 5. If you happen to be the owner of an abdominal board such as is made by the YORK BAR BELL COMPANY, you can perform a wide variety of exercises. This makes it possible to gradually increase the intensity of the exercises as using the inclined board amplifies the effort required. One of the best with the board is to lie with your head at the lower end of the board;

holding the feet together, keeping the legs straight, wave them in circles. Six movements one way and six with the opposite direction of rotation. As your muscles become powerful you can perform this exercise with weights attached to your feet.

No. 6. Take a fairly heavy dumbell in one hand. Extend it perpendicularly overhead. Holding the bell in that position reach down and touch the toe on the same side of the arm holding the weight. By twisting to this opposite side the entire mid-section gets more exercise. Repeat six to twelve times with each arm. After touching toe come back to the straight position, looking to the front but with weight overhead.

No. 7. This exercise of swinging a bar bell can be done in two ways. It is the old army setting-up exercise and a very good one. Of course it exercises the back. But this is necessary as many men find fat collecting on their buttocks and this will help. Others have lumps of fat forming upon the sides of their back. This exercise will help keep it away. The sides and front abdominals get their share of the exercise. Raise the bar bell to arm's length overhead. It should be light enough that it is not too hard for you to handle. Keeping the arms straight, lean over so that the bar just about touches the floor opposite the right foot. Then back to the center position and nearly touch the floor opposite the left foot. Perform this exercise from 6 to 12 times.

No. 8. For really advanced exercise, a Roman chair, Roman column, or even a bench will permit a wide variety of exercises. With either system you have a strap into which you can hold the feet. Holding a bar bell behind neck or at arm's length, using dumbells in the same position or a weight on your chest you go far back, turn and twist the body at all sorts of angles. A marvelously muscled torso will result.

No. 9. One dumbell swing or two dumbell swing. Both are good exercises. If you are to perform this with one dumbell, swing the bell far back between the legs, permitting the knees to bend slightly. Holding the non-lifting hand on the opposite knee and keeping your back as flat as possible you swing the bell up and far back. Perform this exercise rapidly and the abdomen gets its principal work as the body stops and starts down again. Change hands with each movement as the weight reaches the top position. The exercise is performed in much the same manner with two dumbells as it is with one. You will find this a bit harder.

No. 10. This exercise requires considerable agility and strength. If you can learn to do it you can be sure that you will have a slender, well muscled stomach. Lie flat upon the floor. Draw up the legs so that the knees are bent and the feet flat upon the floor. Reach the hands back of head turning them so that the palms will be down. Gradually raise the body pulling the arms and legs together as the waist is raised into the air. You will be standing with the stomach high in the air and the weight of the body resting on the palms and feet. Some men learn to raise in this manner with weights up to three hundred pounds on their abdomens. As you become proficient you can even learn to walk in this crab position and you will be able to stand with the hands and feet almost together, the body forming a circle. It is hard exercise but a mighty good one.

ABDOMINAL CULTURE:

No. 11. Place two boxes so that they will be more than shoulder width apart. Place the feet on a table or high bench, higher than the boxes. Put one hand on either box. Now go down into the floor-dip position. You will find this to be a good exercise as it permits the body to go lower and the muscles to work from extreme contraction to extreme extension. It can be made progressive by placing weights upon the shoulders. While in this position go through the Namaskur exercises as described in the part of the course without apparatus. You will find this to be one of the best body exercises ever devised. It will be a bit hard at first. But you will be well repaid for your efforts.

No. 12. Another swinging exercise and a good one too. Take a bar bell that is easy to handle. Hold it at arm's length overhead. Now move it fairly far to the right, swing it down to the left and up to arm's length. Then down and and to the right and to arm's length. To get the full benefit of this exercise permit the knees to bend considerably. Let the body bend somewhat to the front and when reaching the position with arms overhead lean a bit back to bring the muscles on the front of the body into play. Swing the bell from twelve to twenty-four times. This exercise will go far toward making you strong and well muscled, slender and youthful in appearance and mighty healthy with all your bodily processes working a hundred per cent perfect. Follow these exercises and the advice given here, and you will feel as you never felt before; feel so good that you would have to take something to hold yourself back if you felt any better.

You are not to attempt to perform the 24 exercises at one time. If you only wish to keep fit perform either half or all of the first twelve exercises five times a week. Rest two days of each week.

After you have progressed to a fair extent you can go on to the more advanced exercises and reach the limit of abdominal development and condition.

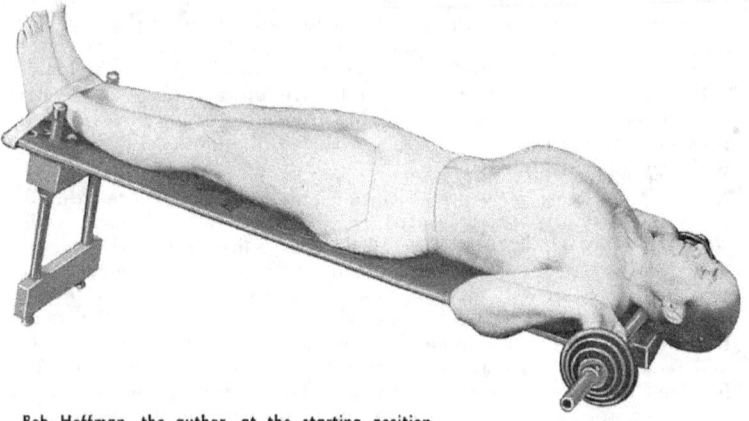

Bob Hoffman, the author, at the starting position of the sit-up exercise on an adjustable York abdominal board.

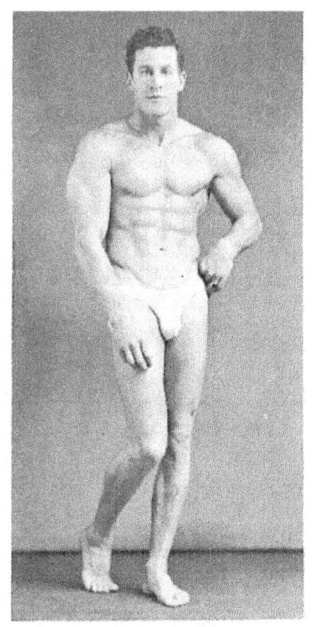

SAMSON DUNLAP

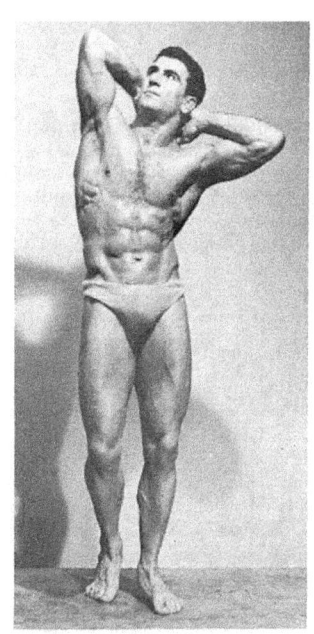

ANDRE DRAPP

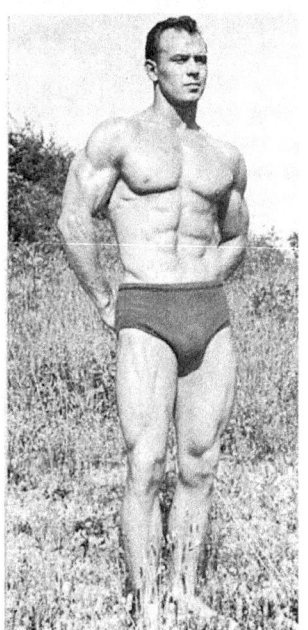

IRVIN KOSZEWSKI

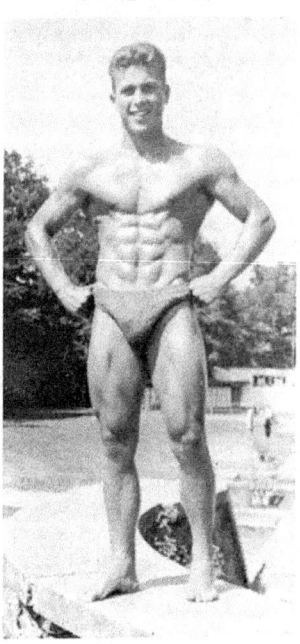

CHARLES KLEJNIAK

Better Health
Through Overcoming Obesity

WEBSTER'S DICTIONARY defines obesity as "An excessive corpulence, especially of an unhealthy kind, excessive fatness of body." The term "obesity," while applied to those who have large fleshy bodies in general, is usually considered to apply chiefly to an oversized waistline.

Look around you and you will note that the vast majority of men and women past thirty-five, or even thirty, have more than generous waistlines. This condition is not only unsightly, but definitely unhealthy as well. A swollen, very fat abdomen is the direct cause of a large percentage of the minor and major bodily ills, for fat, which clings to the surface of the muscles of most sections of the body, is not only upon the surface of the abdomen, but in greater quantity within. This internal fat clogs and hampers the action of every internal organ and gland, handicaps their every action so that many bodily irregularities occur.

It has long been observed that people exercise for two major reasons—to look well and to feel well. And there is no better way to improve one's appearance and one's feelings (really the state of health), than to practice abdominal exercises coupled with some adherence to better diet and improved posture. There are two accepted methods to reduce over-all obesity—diet and exercise. Unfortunately those who have tried diet alone as a means of reducing their too corpulent bodies, their too obese abdominal regions, have found that they lost the weight in the wrong places. The arms and legs become thin almost to the point of emaciation while there is still a too generous deposit of fat around the waistline. This proves the need for exercise as well as diet in reducing. Before a person has lost the objectionable deposits of fat around the mid-section entirely through diet, the diet must be restricted to the point where one's energy and endurance are greatly reduced, and where one's physical reserves reach a dangerously low point, thus placing the dieter in a position where he or she can easily fall prey to many diseases.

It is recognized that certain articles of food have greater fat-producing properties than others, so it is evident that diet—eating less of fat-forming foods—should have a part in overcoming obesity. Fat likes to form in a nice, quiet, undisturbed place. With most people, this section is the abdominal region and the hips and buttocks. People, especially those who like to live well, have a tendency to pet and pamper that corpulent mid-section. As soon as this part of their anatomy becomes swollen and enlarged they seem to believe that they can hurt it easily, so are very cautious in their movements, particularly avoiding bending as much as possible. This doubles or triples the formation of fat until you soon see the individual, man or woman, walking about the street leaning back to balance the greatly oversized waistline, as if he or she were carrying a bass drum.

To overcome obesity and to acquire the superhealth, more pep and endurance which will result, specialized exercise is necessary. Overweight persons need locally applied exercise, intelligently and conscientiously pursued. Don't get frightened and stop reading at this point, you people who are suffering from obesity; you need not go through a protracted siege of "physical torture." There are several comparatively easy ways to reduce your waistline, and thus obtain a new body for the old. If you prefer, every one of these splendid exercises could be practiced lying down, either in bed or upon the floor of your bedroom or living room. It will not detract from your energy or make you a bit uncomfortable, and you will receive a rich reward for your moderate efforts.

You would be right if you regarded obesity as a disease which must be specifically treated like any other disease. When the natural processes of the body are carried out naturally and normally, there will be no unusual accumulation of fat. A little fat is a good thing, but more than five per cent. of surplus fat is dangerous and the more fat you have the more dangerous the condition becomes, so that those who are fifty per cent. overweight have a death rate seventy-four per cent greater than normal. The failing of some natural process invariably results in the rapid formation of fat. Change of life in women particularly and the similar losing of sex power and reduced activity in men are largely responsible for this rapid increase in obesity, unless some effort is made to prevent the formation of fat.

The best means of all to overcome this condition of obesity is specialized exercise, coupled with improved posture, self-administered massage, and at least a moderate reduction of the fat-forming foods which are placed within the body. You need not starve, you need not be uncomfortable; you will receive a rich reward for the moderate efforts you put forth to reduce your waistline, to overcome your obesity.

You need specialized exercise, for exercise directly attacks the superfluous fat and when you practice abdominal movements you are reducing the fat within and without. Fat is rapidly dissipated when a regular habit of exercising the mid-section is adopted. Movements of the muscles which are surrounded with fat quickly break down and dissipate the fatty deposits. Fat is a soft, watery substance. not too resistant to specialized exercise. Special abdominal exercises, coupled with a bit of self-administered massage between exercises, will break down and eliminate fatty deposits with surprising speed, for fat in anything except small quantities will not cling to an active muscle.

Before going on to the real purpose of this article and others of a similar nature which will follow, we will discuss briefly the ills which are a direct result of obesity. Indigestion, dyspepsia and constipation are the names applied to the three major conditions which cause discomfort in the mid-section. While very annoying in themselves, they often lead to many more serious ills. But they provide enough direct discomfort and inconvenience, in themselves, to well make it worth anyone's

while to do everything possible to eliminate them.

When a person says that he has indigestion it may include many forms of abdominal discomfort. It may mean anything from a loss of appetite and a bad taste in the mouth, cramps, mild discomfort to nausea, sick headaches, vomiting and diarrhea, gaseous distention and eructation of gas. This so-called indigestion may be a mild functional disturbance, or the forerunner of a serious disease.

A survey showed that a large percentage of men over forty years of age who complained of indigestion and dyspepsia were found to have ulcers of the stomach, gall bladder disease, or cancer of the gastrointestinal tract or accessory organ. If your troublesome condition persists, you will be wise to consult your family physician and have him seek for your trouble. There are few doctors indeed who do not realize the value of exercise, and who will not recommend exercise to improve your health and physical condition if their diagnosis does not find something very wrong with you, such as cancer, or appendicitis.

But if this pain and discomfort you have occurs only at times, and seems to be the result of overeating and drinking, you know that you can easily overcome this condition in the future. Seventy-five per cent. of American people suffer more or less from constipation, spend over fifty millions of dollars annually to aid their condition, which could be eliminated by more careful attention to diet and to the inclusion of a reasonable amount of specialized exercise in their daily life. While exercise is most important in overcoming constipation, the eating of a normal, well-balanced diet containing a fair share of roughage, fruit and vegetables will help to prevent and overcome the condition. Stewed fruits, notably prunes, will help, as will the habit of going to the toilet regularly; upon arising or after breakfast and other meals are good times. Avoid nervous tension, drink a good quantity of water. Exercises such as will be contained in this series of articles will be most helpful in overcoming this too prevalent condition of constipation.

Your first problem is to get control of your waistline. There are few men and women, regardless of their physical condition and their neglect of the mid-section, who do not have enough control to lift their chests and to pull in their waistlines. If you did nothing in the line of physical exercise except improve your posture and learn to draw in your abdomen, you could reduce your waistline by inches.

One of the very best ways to reduce your abdomen inside and out is this drawing in of the belly every time you think of it during the day. When you find yourself standing or sitting in a bad posture, straighten up, pull in your abdomen. This voluntary contraction of the abdominal muscles can be practiced many times a day. It can be done at any time, any place, when you are walking, sitting, standing or lying down. The movement is more beneficial when it is done solely through the action of the abdominal muscles without expansion of the chest. Without physical effort, be sure that your chest is in the proper position, then draw in your waistline as far as you can. You can draw in, relax, draw in, etc., or you can hold it in for a considerable period in any of the positions mentioned.

This pulling in of the belly does more for you than merely causing a group of muscles to function. First it serves as a reminder of the need for better posture. It provides exercise for the abdominal muscles, making it more difficult for fat to cling to the external muscles. It has an effect on the blood supply of the abdominal organs, for its pump-like action stimulates the circulation and eliminates the stagnation which is too often present in the obese abdominal region, owing to the congestion of poor position and fatty deposits. It has a massaging effect on the internal organs, wears away and breaks up the fat, stimulates the action of the internal organs and glands, strengthens their action, through strengthening the muscues which surround and support them. It stimulates elimination, the action of the bowels, thus playing a major part in overcoming constipation. But its most important result, aside from the strengthening of the muscles, the improvement of the appearance, is the manner in which it aids in the removal of internal fat; for it is an established truth, a physiological law, that the frequent use of muscles in any region causes absorption of fat in that region.

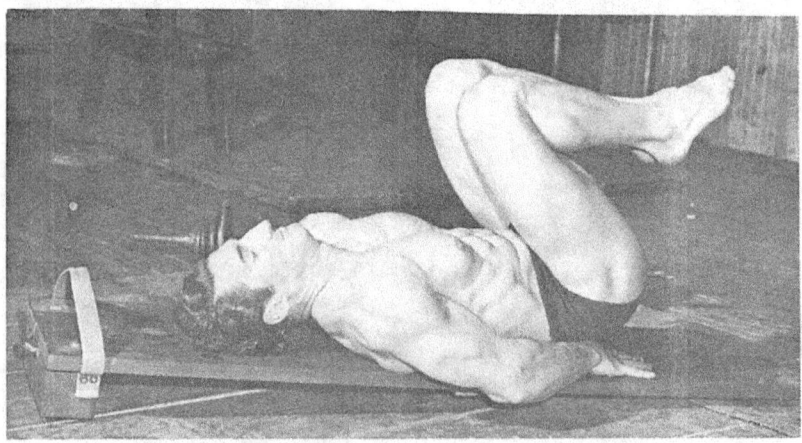

Joe Lauriano of the York Barbell Club, the Jr. Mr. America of 1945 and repeated winner of "Best Abdominals," demonstrates an effective exercise for the mid-section.

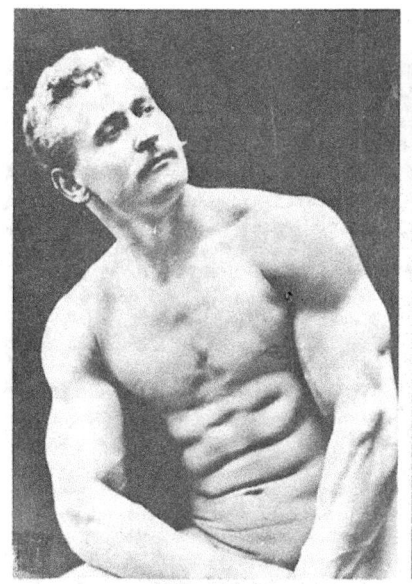

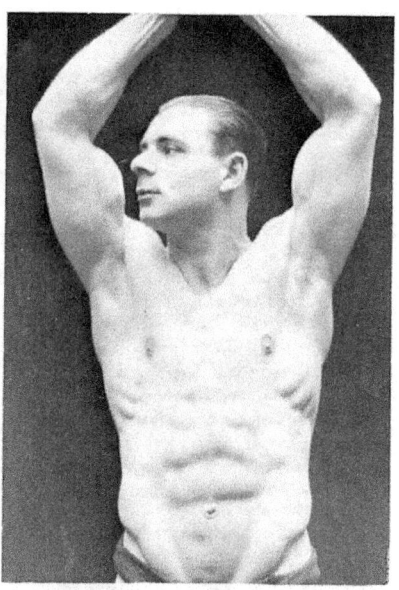

EUGENE SANDOW   SIEGMUND KLEIN

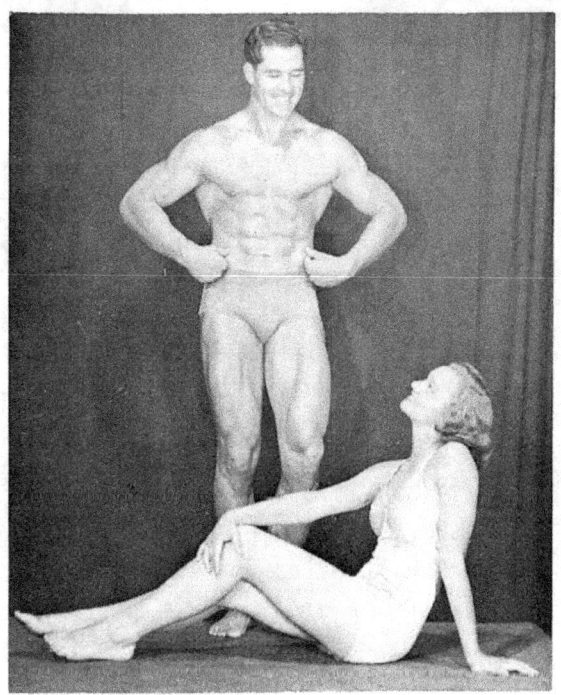

RUTH AUCAMP AND CORRIE PRETORIUS

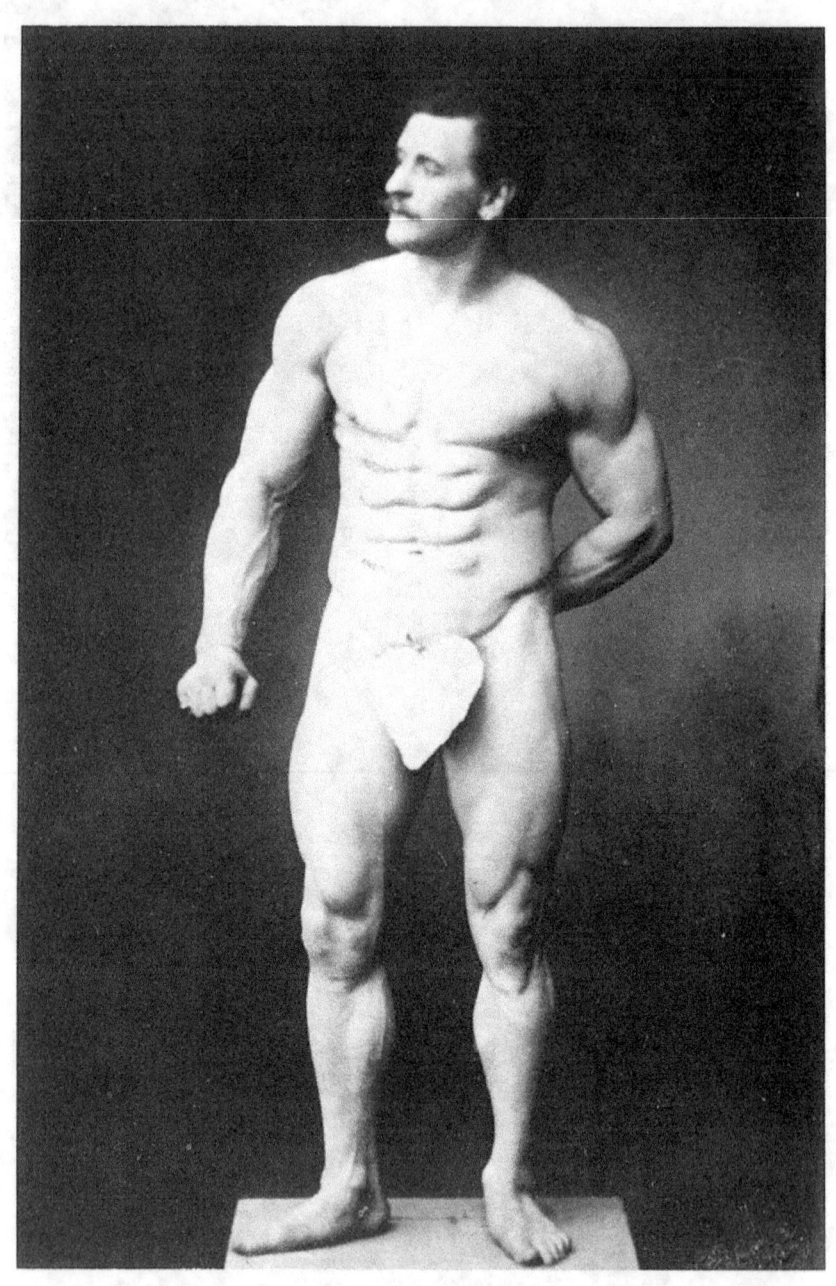

EUGENE SANDOW

York Abdominal Course Exercise Chart

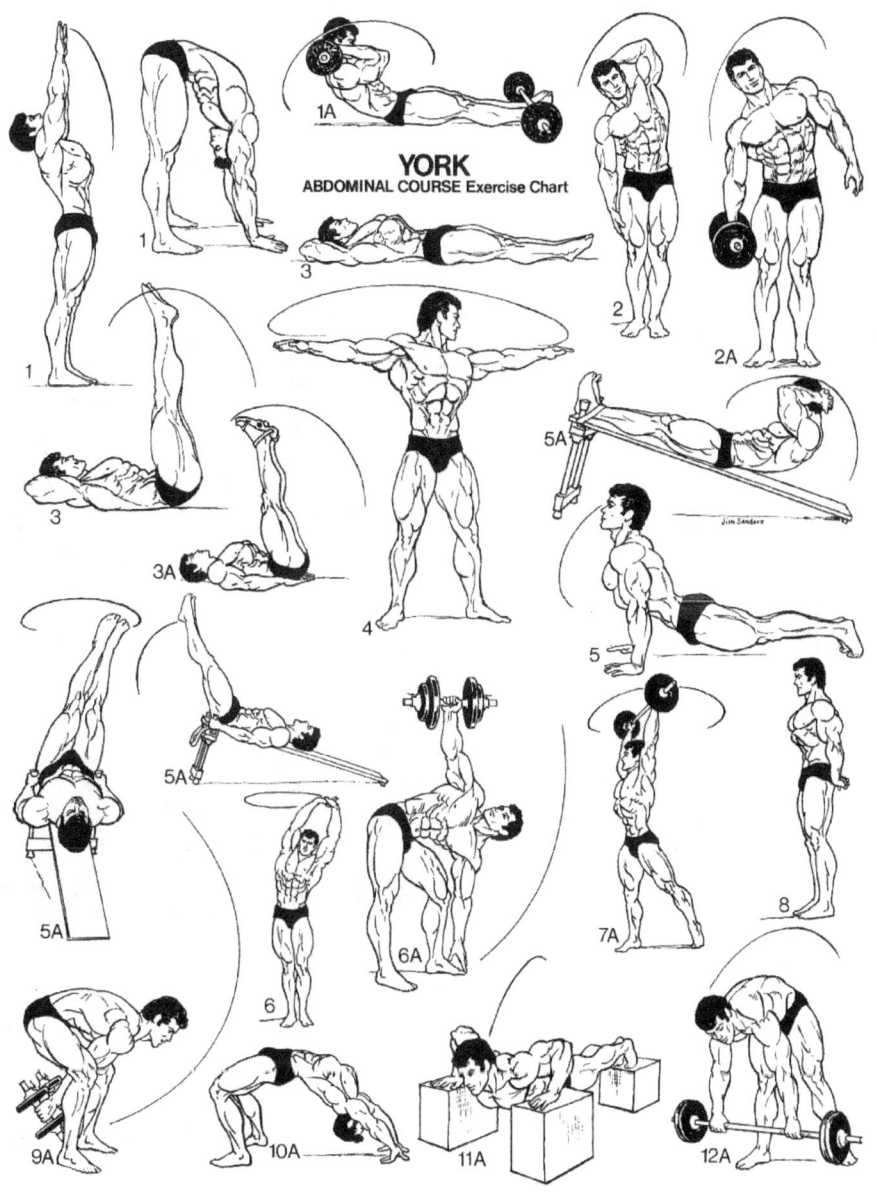

YORK
ABDOMINAL COURSE Exercise Chart

Editor's Biography

Roger is an authority on old time strongman weightlifting techniques. He worked for the York Barbell Company as the Olympic Lifting Advisor. At York, he had access to many original files and people who made York Barbell the "Strongest Name in Fitness." Roger began collecting memorabilia and cataloging the industry's history to preserve these important techniques and stories.

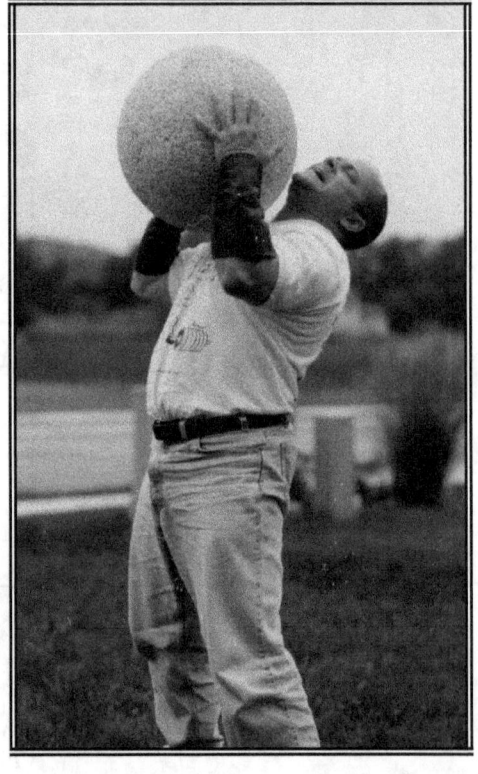

As a weightlifter, Roger has competed in Olympic style weightlifting, powerlifting competitions and All-Round Weightlfting competitions, where he has broken National and World Records in several lifts. He has done this in both the Open Division, as well as Master's Age Divisions in drug free competition. His unique approach to training as a Master's age athlete is bringing more attention to his methods than anyone ever expected.

Articles by and about Roger LaPointe and Atomic Athletic have appeared in Outside Magazine, World Weightlifting, PowerMag, Monster Muscle, Men's Journal, York Daily Record, the Toledo Blade, the Sentinel-Tribune, and numerous other publications.

Roger has also been interviewed for television and radio. The list of web sites that have included articles, references and photos is too numerous to list.

Roger can be contacted for consultation and speaking engagements through his website at www.atomicathletic.com.

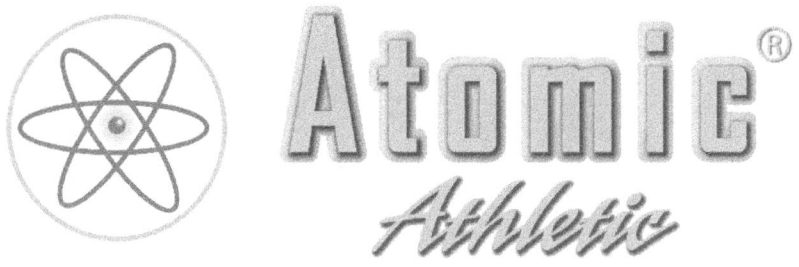

AtomicAthletic.com

MORE OUTSTANDING OLD TIME STRONGMAN &
TRADITIONAL STRENGTH TRAINING PUBLICATIONS
BY ROGER LaPOINTE

Garage Gym Guide
Traditional Training Legendary Strength
Train Like a Strongman
Leg Development
Stone Lifting Special Reports
Ankle Stability Kit
Atomic Athletic Bomb Proof Bulletins Compiled Vol. 1

New Editions
Gymnastique Digitale: Finger Gymnastics by Adolphe Roche*
Light Dumb-Bell Exercises

*This is printed in three languages in this single publication.

www.ingramcontent.com/pod-product-compliance
Lightning Source LLC
Chambersburg PA
CBHW070457290526
45791CB00005B/2150